The New MRCPsych Paper III Practice MCQs and EMIs

OLIVER WHITE

BMedSci, BM BS, MRCPsych

Specialist Registrar in Child and Adolescent and Forensic Psychiatry, Oxford Deanery

and

CLARE OAKLEY

MB ChB, MRCPsych

Specialty Registrar in Forensic Psychiatry, West Midlands Deanery

Radcliffe Publishing
Oxford • New York

Radcliffe Publishing Ltd
18 Marcham Road
Abingdon
Oxon OX14 1AA
United Kingdom

www.radcliffe-oxford.com
Electronic catalogue and worldwide online ordering facility.

British Library Cataloguing in Publication Data

A catalogue record for this book is available from the British Library.

ISBN-13: 978 184619 255 5

Typeset by Pindar NZ, Auckland, New Zealand
Printed and bound by TJI Digital, Padstow, Cornwall, UK

Contents

About the authors

Oliver White graduated in 2001 and worked in Nottingham and Sydney, Australia prior to completing his basic psychiatric training on the Mid Trent rotation. He is currently an SpR dual training in Child and Adolescent and Forensic Psychiatry in the Oxford Deanery. Oliver developed an interest in training issues as an SHO and for the past three years has been a member of the Psychiatric Trainees' Committee of the Royal College of Psychiatrists and is currently Chair of the Committee. He is therefore experienced in the recent changes in psychiatric training, including the development of the new MRCPsych exams.

Clare Oakley graduated from the University of Birmingham in 2003 and undertook her basic psychiatric training in Birmingham. She is currently a Specialty Registrar in Forensic Psychiatry in the West Midlands Deanery. Clare has been a member of the Psychiatric Trainees' Committee of the Royal College of Psychiatrists for the last two years and is currently its Vice Chair. She is involved in developing the curriculum and workplace-based assessments within the Royal College of Psychiatrists and so has an extensive knowledge of the assessment system, including the new MRCPsych exams.

Introduction

Background

The structure of the MRCPsych examination has changed significantly. The exam will no longer consist of two distinct parts but will consist of three written papers and one clinical exam. This chapter outlines these changes, and further details can be found on the website of the Royal College of Psychiatrists (www.rcpsych.ac.uk). We recommend that candidates check the website carefully before applying to sit the examinations. This book provides 250 practice MCQs and 100 practice EMIs for paper III.

Examination format

The new written papers will contain 200 questions and will all be three hours long. The papers will include both 'single best answer 1 from 5' style MCQs, and EMIs. The proportion of each type of question in the exam paper may vary but approximately one-third of the questions will be EMIs.

There will be a new OSCE-type examination called Clinical Assessment of Skills and Competencies (CASC). It will consist of two parts to be completed in one day. One circuit will consist of eight individual stations of seven minutes with a preceding one-minute 'preparation' time. The other circuit will consist of four pairs of linked stations, with the stations each lasting ten minutes, with two minutes of preparation time.

Examination content

The topics tested in each paper are shown in the table below. Broadly speaking, paper I can be considered to be similar to the old Part 1 written paper; paper II has elements similar to the Part 2 basic sciences paper; paper III is similar to the Part 2 clinical sciences paper with additional critical appraisal and statistics.

Paper I	Paper II	Paper III
History and mental state examination	General principles of psychopharmacology (pharmacokinetics, pharmacodynamics)	Research methods
Cognitive assessment		Evidence-based practice
Neurological examination	Psychotropic drugs	Statistics
Assessment	Adverse reactions	Critical appraisal
Aetiology	Evaluation of treatments	Clinical topics
Diagnosis	Neurosciences (physiology, endocrinology, chemistry, anatomy, pathology)	General adult
Classification		Liaison
Basic psychopharmacology		Forensic
Basic psychological processes	Genetics	Addiction
Social psychology	Statistics and research (basic)	Child and adolescent
Description and measurement	Epidemiology	Psychotherapy
Basic psychological treatments	Advanced psychological processes and treatments	Learning disability
Human psychological development		Rehabilitation
Descriptive psychopathology		Old age psychiatry
Dynamic psychopathology		
Prevention of psychiatric disorder		
History of psychiatry		
Basic ethics and philosophy of psychiatry		
Stigma and culture		

The proportion of questions in each topic in the chapters of this book is based on the indicative breakdown of questions provided by the College.

Techniques for answering questions
MCQs

- Read the question carefully.
- Watch out for double negatives.
- Narrow down the five options by first excluding those that you know are incorrect.
- Phrases that include 'can' 'may' and 'is possible' are often true.
- Phrases that include 'always' 'never' and 'essential' are often false.
- Understand what the following terms mean:
    - characteristic: you would doubt the diagnosis without this
    - typical: same as characteristic
    - pathognomonic: occurs in that disease and no other
    - specific: same as pathognomonic
    - recognised: this has been reported
    - commonly: more than 50%
    - rare: less than 5%
    - almost never: 1–2%.

EMIs

Each option may be used once, more than once, or not at all. Each question may have more than one answer (this will be indicated). It may be helpful to read the question first before reading the answer options. EMIs take longer than MCQs to answer – make sure you allow enough time.

Recommended reading

Candidates will have their own preferences about textbooks and revision material. We found the following books useful in our preparation for the Membership exams and they cover most of the material required. In the explanatory notes that accompany the answers in this book, there are references to the books below to enable you to read more fully if you have not understood a topic.

Fear C. *Essential Revision Notes in Psychiatry for MRCPsych*. Knutsford: PasTest; 2004.

Johnstone E, Cunningham-Owens DG, Lawrie SM, *et al.*, editors. *Companion to Psychiatric Studies*. 7th ed. London: Churchill Livingstone; 2004.

Lawrie SM, McIntosh AM, Rao S. *Critical Appraisal for Psychiatry*. Edinburgh: Elsevier Churchill Livingstone; 2000.

Leung WC, Passmore K. *Essential Notes in Basic Sciences for the MRCPsych Part 2*. Oxford: Radcliffe Publishing; 2004.

Levi MI. *Basic Notes in Psychiatry*. 4th ed. Oxford: Radcliffe Publishing; 2005.

Puri BK, Hall AD. *Revision Notes in Psychiatry*. 2nd revised ed. London: Hodder Arnold; 2004.

Semple D, Smyth R, Burns J, *et al. Oxford Handbook of Psychiatry*. Oxford: Oxford University Press; 2005.

Stone JH, Roberts M, O'Grady J, *et al. Faulk's Basic Forensic Psychiatry*. 3rd ed. Oxford: Blackwell Publishing; 2000.

Taylor D, Paton C, Kerwin R. *The Maudsley 2005–2006 Prescribing Guidelines*. 8th ed. Abingdon: Taylor & Francis; 2005.

2

Critical appraisal

Questions

MCQs

The following information should be considered when answering questions 1 to 7.

A questionnaire for detecting anxiety was developed to be filled in by patients in primary care. A study was conducted in which 425 consecutive patients attending three inner city general practices were asked to complete the questionnaire and were then interviewed by the researchers. The results are shown in the table below.

Anxiety questionnaire	Structured diagnostic interview		
	Anxiety disorder diagnosed	No anxiety disorder diagnosed	Total
Anxiety diagnosed	39	103	142
Anxiety not diagnosed	6	277	283
Total	45	380	425

1 The prevalence of anxiety disorders in the study is:
   a 1%
   b 11%
   c 5%
   d 9%
   e 3%

2 The sensitivity of the anxiety questionnaire is:
  a 28%
  b 73%
  c 52%
  d 87%
  e 98%

3 The specificity of the anxiety questionnaire is:
  a 98%
  b 87%
  c 48%
  d 28%
  e 73%

4 The positive predictive value of the anxiety questionnaire is:
  a 48%
  b 28%
  c 87%
  d 73%
  e 37%

5 The negative predictive value of the anxiety questionnaire is:
  a 11%
  b 28%
  c 98%
  d 87%
  e 66%

6 The likelihood ratio of a positive test is:
  a 1.4
  b 3.2
  c 5.6
  d 9.3
  e 14

7 The questionnaire is:

a Good at correctly diagnosing anxiety

b A useful diagnostic tool

c Good at correctly identifying those who do not have anxiety

d Able to discriminate between different types of anxiety

e Useful for screening patients in a psychiatric clinic

The following information should be considered when answering questions 8 to 11.

A study was undertaken to assess the risk factors for development of antisocial personality disorder (ASPD). A group of 347 10-year-old children underwent a variety of assessments, including the detecting of conduct disorder or attention-deficit hyperactivity disorder (ADHD) and IQ testing. Fifteen years later they were assessed to establish the presence of ASPD. The following results were found:

	ASPD in adulthood	No ASPD in adulthood
Conduct disorder in childhood	57	290
No conduct disorder in childhood	32	313

	Odds ratio	95% confidence interval
Low IQ	1.2	0.74–1.36
ADHD	1.6	1.27–1.81

8 What type of study is this?

a Case-control study

b Randomised control trial

c Ecological study

d Cohort study

e Qualitative study

9 What is the odds ratio of having ASPD if there was conduct disorder in childhood?

a 0.2

b 0.5

c 0.9

d 1.6

e 1.9

10 Which of the following statements about confidence intervals is false?

a They are the range within which the true measure actually lies

b They give the same information as p values

c They are a measure of dispersion of data

d They give the precision of a measure

e A narrow confidence interval allows more confidence in the results

11 What is the most accurate summary of the findings of the study?

a Conduct disorder in childhood is the only risk factor for ASPD in adulthood

b Conduct disorder, ADHD and low IQ are all risk factors for developing ASPD

c No risk factors for ASPD have been identified

d Conduct disorder and ADHD are the only risk factors for developing ADHD

e Insufficient information is provided

The following information should be considered when answering questions 12 to 19.

A study was conducted to evaluate the effectiveness of a newly developed mood stabiliser in acute mania. Patients with a diagnosis of mania who were aged between 18 and 65 were included. Patients who had a serious medical condition, had a history of side effects with lithium, were pregnant or abused substances were excluded.

Patients did not know which treatment they would get and were assigned by block randomisation to the new drug, lithium or placebo, which were given in flexible dosage for 21 days. Changes in dosage were made by a clinician who was not involved with allocation or assessing outcome. Recovery was defined as the patient having a reduction of 50% in their score on a rating scale of symptoms in mania.

The baseline characteristics of the patients in the three groups were comparable. All randomised patients were included in the analysis on an intention-to-treat basis. Recovery occurred in 39% of the new drug group, 47% of the lithium group and 25% of the placebo group.

12 What type of study is this?
   a Double-blind randomised control trial
   b Meta-analysis
   c Single-blind randomised control trial
   d Single-blind placebo-controlled randomised trial
   e Double-blind placebo-controlled randomised trial

13 Why were pregnant patients excluded from the study?
   a It would be unethical to randomise them
   b They would not be able to cooperate with the study protocol
   c They may react differently to medication
   d They would be too likely to drop out of the study if they went into labour
   e It was not possible to find any pregnant patients who were manic

14 Why is there a lithium arm to the study?
   a To increase the power of the study
   b For patients who cannot tolerate the side effects of the new drug
   c To allow comparison with the gold standard
   d To facilitate patient choice
   e To allow more patients to be recruited

15 What is the purpose of an intention-to-treat analysis?
   a To simplify the analysis
   b To reduce bias caused by drop-outs
   c To stop patients changing treatment during the study
   d To reduce confounding
   e To allow use of parametric statistics

16 What is the absolute benefit of the new drug compared with placebo?
   a 8%
   b 11%
   c 14%
   d 19%
   e 22%

17 What is the absolute benefit of lithium compared with placebo?
   a 8%
   b 11%
   c 14%
   d 19%
   e 22%

18 What is the number needed to treat for the new drug compared with placebo?
   a 4.5
   b 5.3
   c 7.1
   d 9
   e 12.5

19 What is the number needed to treat for lithium compared with placebo?
   a 4.5
   b 5.3
   c 7.1
   d 9
   e 12.5

20 What is the best summary of the results of this study?
   a The study design is too flawed to draw any conclusions
   b The new drug is more effective than lithium
   c The new drug is no more effective than placebo
   d The new drug is less effective than lithium
   e There is no difference between the effectiveness of the new drug and lithium

21 Which of the following does not minimise the effect of confounding?
   a Blinding
   b Restricting the study population
   c Matching
   d Stratification
   e Multivariate analysis

22 Which method can be used to evaluate the possibility of publication bias in a meta-analysis?
   a Funnel plot
   b F statistic
   c Confidence interval of the summary effect size
   d Log rank test
   e P value of the summary effect size

23 Specificity is:

    a The proportion of people with the disorder who have a positive test

    b The probability of a positive test coming from someone with a disorder compared to someone without the disorder

    c The proportion of people with a positive test who actually have the disorder

    d The proportion of people with a negative test who do not have the disorder

    e The proportion of people without the disorder who have a negative test

24 Which of the following reduces bias?

    a Block randomisation

    b Intention to treat

    c Stratification

    d Minimisation

    e Regression methods

For questions 25 to 27 please read the following précis.

There is a well-established depression scale (A) with 100 items and a new scale (B) with 12 items. Scale B only takes 10 minutes to administer. Both scales A and B were administered to 100 depressed inpatients and 100 controls. Spearman's correlation r = 0.8 p < 0.01. High scores on A correlated with high scores on B.

25 Which of the following is true?

    a A and B are highly linearly correlated

    b A is a good screening tool

    c B is a good measure of depression

    d B can replace A

    e A and B show good inter-rater reliability

26 Which of the following statements about Spearman's correlation coefficient is false?

    a It converts raw values to ranks

b It measures association

c The values will lie between −1 and +1

d It is a parametric test

e It tends to inflate the strength of the association when there are many tied values

27 Which of the following is true?

a Because A is longer than B it must be better

b A is more valid than B

c B is more valid than A

d B is more reliable than A

e We have not been given enough information to assess reliability

28 Which of the following is a test for parametric data?

a *t*-test

b Wilcoxon

c Chi-squared test

d Spearman's rank

e Mann-Whitney U-test

29 Sensitivity is:

a The proportion of people with the disorder who have a positive test

b The probability of a positive test coming from someone with a disorder compared to someone without the disorder

c The proportion of people with a positive test who actually have the disorder

d The proportion of people with a negative test who do not have the disorder

e The proportion of people without the disorder who have a negative test

30 What is kappa score a measure of?

    a Internal consistency

    b Criterion validity

    c Inter-rater reliability

    d Construct validity

    e Test-retest reliability

31 If you wish to consider the effectiveness of an antidepressant, which is the best source of evidence?

    a Expert opinion

    b Randomised control trial

    c Systematic review

    d Meta-analysis

    e Local clinical guideline

32 The following is a description of which statistical test: it compares expected with observed frequencies and is distribution-free?

    a *t*-test

    b Wilcoxon

    c Chi-squared test

    d Spearman's rank

    e Mann-Whitney U-test

33 In meta-analysis, what is meant by clinical heterogeneity?

    a The results of different studies differ from one another significantly more than would be expected by chance

    b The methodologies of the studies are significantly different

    c The subjects in different studies differ from one another significantly

    d It is not possible to combine the results in a meta-analysis

    e The studies used different methods of statistical analysis

34 The quality-adjusted-life-year could be used in which type of economic analysis?

    a Cost minimisation

    b Cost-benefit

    c Cost-effectiveness

    d Cost-utility

    e It would not be used

35 Which of these statements about ANOVA is false?

    a It considers between-groups and within-groups variance

    b It is a parametric test

    c It tests the null hypothesis that the mean values of three or more independent groups are equal

    d The test statistic is F

    e It has an equivalent called the Mann-Whitney U-test

36 Which of the following is not an advantage of cohort studies?

    a They are ethically safe

    b It is possible to calculate incident rates from the results

    c Subjects are matched

    d They are relatively quick to complete

    e It is possible to examine many outcomes for a single exposure

37 Which of the following is the correct definition for internal validity?

    a Internal consistency in construction (similar questions correlate well)

    b Integrity of experimental design

    c Appropriateness of applying results to non-study populations

    d Whether a test appears to be valid

    e The test improves on decisions made from existing information or simpler techniques

38 Which of the following is not true about confidence intervals?

a The intervals are larger with smaller sample size

b They indicate the presence or otherwise of a statistical difference between two groups

c A 95% confidence interval means that 95% of all observed values fall within that interval

d In an odds ratio, if the 95% confidence interval includes unity then no significant difference may apply

e The intervals give a range of values within which the true value will lie

39 Which of the following statements about non-parametric tests is not true?

a They can be applied to ordinal data

b They can be used to analyse samples that are normally distributed

c They can be used on small samples

d Student's paired *t*-test is a non-parametric test

e They can be used if the nature of the distribution of the data is unknown

40 In statistics, which of the following is true?

a The null hypothesis describes the probability that a relationship exists between two samples

b Skewed data invalidates further statistical analysis

c Descriptive statistical tests that measure range include mean, median and mode

d The mode is the measurement that lies exactly between each end of a range of values ranked in order

e Analytical statistics are the same as inferential statistics

41 Regarding the Pearson product-moment correlation coefficient, which of the following is false?

a It is measured on a scale of 0 to 1

b It is denoted by the symbol 'r'

c It describes the degree of agreement between two variables d Positive value implies that a rise in one variable accompanies a rise in the other

  e Ideally, there should be at least 30 subjects per group for a valid calculation

For questions 42 to 51 please refer to the following information.

Developments in functional neuroimaging have lead to the development of a diagnostic MRI scan for early-onset schizophrenia. The accuracy of this scan was tested, with the following results:

	Subjects with schizophrenia	Subjects without schizophrenia	Total
Schizophrenia diagnosed via MRI	228	24	252
Schizophrenia not diagnosed via MRI	13	135	148
Total	241	159	400

42 What is the number of false positives in this sample?
  a 228
  b 24
  c 61
  d 252
  e 289

43 What is the sensitivity of the MRI scan as a diagnostic test?
  a 0.85
  b 0.15
  c 0.05
  d 0.95
  e 0.60

44 What is the specificity of the MRI scan as a diagnostic test?

a 0.59

b 0.05

c 0.10

d 0.95

e 0.85

45 What is the positive predictive value?

a 0.90

b 0.85

c 0.95

d 0.91

e 0.63

46 What is the negative predictive value?

a 0.95

b 0.63

c 0.91

d 0.90

e 0.85

47 What is the likelihood ratio of a positive test?

a 17

b 6.33

c 0.16

d 1.12

e 19

48 What is the pre-test probability?

a 0.63

b 0.37

c 0.34

d 0.60

e 0.57

49 What are the pre-test odds?

   a 0.60

   b 0.89

   c 1.5

   d 1.12

   e 0.67

50 What are the post-test odds?

   a 1.42

   b 7.45

   c 0.40

   d 4.24

   e 6.01

51 What is the post-test probability?

   a 0.81

   b 0.85

   c 1.24

   d 0.88

   e 0.86

For questions 52 to 59 please refer to the following information.

A study investigated the efficacy of a new antidepressant, 'drug X'. There were 2074 depressed subjects recruited into the study and randomly prescribed to either drug X or to the established anti-depressant venlafaxine for a period of 12 weeks. Improvement in mood was measured via the Hamilton Depression Rating Scale (HAM-D). Results are shown below:

	Improvement in HAM-D score	No improvement in HAM-D score	Total
Venlafaxine	684	368	1052
Drug X	707	315	1022
Total	1391	683	2074

52 What type of study is this?

  a Cohort study

  b Qualitative study

  c Randomised control trial

  d Case-control study

  e Ecological study

53 What is the experimental event rate (EER)?

  a 0.31

  b 0.69

  c 0.51

  d 0.35

  e 0.75

54 What is the control event rate (CER)?

  a 0.35

  b 0.51

  c 0.31

  d 0.69

  e 0.65

55 What is the absolute benefit increase (ABI)?

  a 4%

  b 34%

   c 10%

   d 7%

   e 18%

56 What is the relative risk (RR)?

   a 1.12

   b 0.94

   c 1.97

   d 1.06

   e 0.78

57 Patients prescribed drug X are how many more times likely to improve compared than patients prescribed venlafaxine?

   a 0.12

   b 0.22

   c 0.06

   d 0.97

   e 1.04

58 How many patients need to be given drug X in order to prevent one failure to improve on HAM-D score if treated with venlafaxine?

   a 4 patients

   b 12 patients

   c 20 patients

   d 40 patients

   e 25 patients

59 What is the generally accepted number needed to treat (NNT) that is regarded as clinically significant?

   a < 4

   b < 8

   c < 10

   d < 25

   e < 40

60 Which of the following is a feature of the cost-benefit method of economic analysis?

a Costs are related to a clinical output measure

b Outputs are assumed equal

c QALYs are often used

d Inputs and outputs are measured in monetary terms

e Only the inputs are considered

61 New entrants to a multinational organisation are all given a routine medical examination in which three of the recorded variates are age in years, weight in kilograms and colour of eyes. Respectively, these variates are:

a Qualitative, discrete, discrete

b Quantitative, discrete, discrete

c Quantitative, continuous, discrete

d Qualitative, discrete, qualitative

e Discrete, continuous, qualitative

62 A truly random sample of the general population would be obtained by which of the following?

a Closing one's eyes and sticking a pin into a telephone directory

b Selecting every individual with a surname beginning with the letter 'S'

c Selecting every twentieth individual from a list of patients registered with a GP

d Allocating each individual a unique number and using a computer to randomly generate numbers for selection

e Selecting an individual from every fourth house on a street

63 In a prospective study of borderline personality disorder following childhood sexual abuse, borderline personality disorder was found in 41 out of 119 subjects (34.5%, 95% CI 25.91% to 42.99%). Which of the following statements is true?

a In the population of individuals who have experienced childhood sexual abuse, the true rate of borderline personality disorder is greater than 34.5%

b In this sample, the rate of borderline personality disorder could take any value between 25.91% and 42.99%

c The true rate of borderline personality disorder in the population of individuals who have experienced childhood sexual abuse is unlikely to be less than 25.91%

d The investigators would have obtained a more precise estimate of the proportion of individuals with borderline personality disorder if they had calculated a 99% confidence interval

e If an earlier study into the same issue had reported that the rate of borderline personality disorder after childhood sexual abuse was only 27.0%, we could conclude that the rate of borderline personality disorder was increasing

64 Which of the following statements is false?

a A meta-analysis concerns the statistical analysis of a very large data set from a clinical trial or observational study

b A meta-analysis is separate from a systematic review

c A meta-analysis can use a forest plot to determine whether the results from the separate studies are compatible and assess the significance of the individual and overall effects

d A meta-analysis has results that are statistically heterogeneous if there is considerable variation between the estimates of the effects of interest from the various studies

e A meta-analysis has results that are clinically heterogeneous if each of the separate studies is focusing on different clinical end points of interest

65 Regarding the cost-effectiveness method of economic analysis, which of the following is true?

a It is not possible to distinguish between interventions providing more benefit at greater cost and interventions providing less benefit at lower cost

b Outputs are assumed equal

c All costs are converted into monetary terms

d Outputs are converted into quality of life measures

e Qualitative and quantitative information is used

For questions 66 to 68 please refer to the following information.

A study was conducted to examine the relationship between alcohol intake and self-harm behaviour. The records of 834 consecutive attendees who presented at a busy A&E department were reviewed and details of alcohol intake over the past week and presentation following an episode of self-harm were recorded. Results are shown in the table below:

	Self-harm behaviour	No self-harm behaviour	Total
Intake of 35 units or greater of alcohol per week	51	42	93
Intake of less than 35 units of alcohol per week	113	628	741
Total	164	670	834

66 What type of study is this?
   a Randomised control trial
   b Cohort study
   c Economic analysis
   d Case-control study
   e Systematic review

67 What is the odds ratio?
   a 4.58
   b 6.75
   c 12.30
   d 2.87
   e 0.34

68 Which of the following types of bias is less likely to be present in the study?

   a Recall bias

   b Information bias

   c Selection bias

   d Interviewer bias

   e Sampling bias

69 Regarding longitudinal studies, which of the following is false?

   a They cannot be used to estimate the incidence of a disease

   b They are either experimental or observational

   c They are not suitable for estimating the point prevalence of a condition

   d They can be used for assessing causality

   e They are either prospective or retrospective

70 Which of the following is true of the p value?

   a It is the probability of obtaining the observed or more extreme results if the alternative hypothesis is true

   b It is the probability that the alternative hypothesis is true

   c It is the probability of obtaining the observed results or results which are more extreme if the null hypothesis is true

   d It is always less than 0.05

   e It is the probability that the null hypothesis is true

71 Regarding the relative risk of a disease, which of the following is true?

   a It measures the risk of the disease in the population

   b It takes the value zero when the risk is equally likely in those exposed and unexposed to the factor of interest

   c It measures the increased (or decreased) risk of the factor when the individual has the disease

   d It always lies between zero and one

   e It is always positive

72 Which of the following is true regarding the power of a test?
   a   It is greater if the effect of interest is smaller than if it is larger
   b   It increases as the variability of the observations decreases
   c   It increases as the significance level decreases
   d   It is the chance of rejecting the null hypothesis when it is true
   e   It decreases as the size of the sample increases

73 In which of the following situations is the one-sample t-test appropriate?
   a   When the variable of interest is categorical
   b   When the aim is to compare the mean of a variable in one group of individuals to that of another
   c   When the variable of interest is not normally distributed
   d   When the assumptions underlying the sign test are not satisfied
   e   When the aim is to compare the mean of a variable in a group of individuals to a particular value

74 Regarding the odds ratio, which of the following is true?
   a   It is equal to zero when the odds of being a case in the exposed and unexposed groups are equal
   b   It is calculated in a case-control study because the relative risk cannot be estimated directly
   c   It is the ratio of the probability of being a case in the exposed group to the probability of not being a case in the exposed group
   d   It is an estimate of the relative risk when the incidence of the disease is common
   e   It cannot be negative

75 The presence of bias in a study implies which of the following?
   a   The results of the study are not precise
   b   There is a systematic difference between the results obtained and those expected
   c   The results of the study are not accurate

d The individuals in the study must have been selected using a random selection procedure

e There are missing readings

EMIs

1 Study designs

a Case-control study

b Open label randomised control trial

c Prospective cohort study

d Ecological study

e Systematic review

f Cross-sectional survey

g Crossover randomised control trial

h Meta-analysis

i Qualitative study

What would be the most ethical type of study to select for the following scenarios:

1 To look at the number of completed suicides in the 12 months following an overdose in people without a mental illness

2 To look at the number of children developing cardiac abnormalities when their mother took lithium during pregnancy

3 To look at obstetric complications and the development of schizophrenia while avoiding attrition bias

4 To look for exposure and outcome while avoiding recall bias

5 To compare treatment to placebo in a situation where the researchers wish to recruit fewer participants

6 To compare whether a new drug has fewer side effects than another established drug

7 To get patients' perspectives on the quality of care they receive

2 Statistical tests
   a Paired *t*-test
   b Chi-squared test
   c Multiple regression
   d McNemar test
   e ANOVA
   f Independent *t*-test
   g Logistic regression
   h Mann-Whitney U-test
   i Pearson product-moment correlation
   j Bonferroni correction
   k Kruskal-Wallis test
   l Spearman's rank correlation
   m Kappa

Which is the most appropriate statistical test?

   1 When measuring the degree of agreement between two independent raters of a variable

   2 When comparing the mean values of more than two groups

   3 When measuring the differences in median results of two independent groups

3 **Screening**
   a 22%
   b 28%
   c 33%
   d 44%
   e 55%
   f 66%
   g 74%
   h 78%
   i 85%

Terminally ill people are screened for depression with the question 'Do you think you are depressed?' This response is then compared to a structured diagnostic interview used to diagnose depression.

Screening question	Structured diagnostic interview		
	Depression diagnosed	No depression diagnosed	Total
Depression diagnosed	11	9	20
No depression diagnosed	14	40	54
Total	25	49	74

1 What was the prevalence of depression in the sample?

2 What was the sensitivity of the screening?

3 What was the specificity of the screening?

4 What proportion of those who screened positive were depressed?

5 What proportion of those who were depressed screened positive?

6 What was the negative predictive value?

4 Study designs
   a Case-control study
   b Double-blind randomised control trial
   c Cohort study
   d Ecological study
   e Systematic review
   f Cross-sectional study
   g Single-blind randomised control trial
   h Meta-analysis
   i Qualitative study

Which type of studies are described below?

1 A study of the whole population using computerised records to generate a hypothesis

2 A statistical review of available evidence from multiple sources

3 An observational analytic comparison of subjects with and without a particular disorder

4 Some patients receive 12 sessions of supportive psychotherapy and some patients receive 12 sessions of CBT

5 Statistical tests
   a Paired *t*-test
   b Chi-squared test
   c Cluster analysis
   d ANOVA
   e Independent *t*-test
   f Linear regression
   g Mann-Whitney U-test
   h Pearson product-moment correlation
   i Bonferroni correction
   j Kruskal-Wallis test
   k Spearman's rank correlation coefficient
   l Standard deviation
   m McNemar test

Match the following descriptions with the statistical tests above:

1 Compares two groups of paired binary data

2 Compares four groups of parametric data

3 Compares two independent groups of normally distributed data

    4 Parametric test that measures the observed association between two variables

    5 Measures the difference between two unpaired sets of categorical data

    6 Compares two unpaired sets of ranked data

6 Biases
- a Publication bias
- b Recall bias
- c Sampling bias
- d Observer bias
- e Information bias
- f Responder bias
- g Measurement bias

Match the situations below with the types of bias listed above.

    1 Recruitment of patients for a study into the side effects of antidementia medication is advertised on the internet.

    2 Patients with opiate dependence are asked about a history of childhood sexual abuse.

    3 A study of hospital inpatients aims to investigate whether split doses of medication lead to reduced side effects.

Answers

MCQs

1 b

45/425 = 10.6%

2 d

39/45 = 86.7%

3 e

277/380 = 72.9%

4 b

39/142 = 27.5%

5 c

277/283 = 97.8%

6 b

0.87/1 – 0.73 = 3.2

7 c

8 d

9 e

Odds ratio (OR) = 57/32 divided by 290/313 = 1.78/0.93 = 1.9

10 b

They give all the information of a p value plus the precision of any estimate (Lawrie, McIntosh, Rao, p. 62).

11 e

No confidence interval for the odds ratio for conduct disorder is provided, so it is not known whether it is statistically significant.

12 e

13 a

Due to the known teratogenic effects of lithium, it would be unethical to randomise them to the lithium arm of the study.

14 c

15 b

16 c

Absolute benefit increase (ABI) = experimental event rate (EER) – control event rate (CER)

ABI = 0.39 – 0.25 = 0.14 = 14%

17 e

ABI = EER – CER

ABI = 0.47 – 0.25 = 0.22 = 22%

18 c

Number needed to treat (NNT) = 1/ABI = 1/0.14 = 7.1

19 a

NNT = 1/ABI = 1/0.22 = 4.5

20 d

21 a

22 a

23 e

24 b

25 c

26 d

It is a distribution-free test (Johnstone, Cunningham-Owens, Lawrie, *et al.*, p. 197).

27 e

28 a

29 a

30 c

(Johnstone, Cunningham-Owens, Lawrie, *et al.*, p. 186)

31 c

32 c

(Johnstone, Cunningham-Owens, Lawrie, *et al.*, p. 194)

33 c

34 d

(Lawrie, McIntosh, Rao, p. 37)

35 e

The non-parametric equivalent of ANOVA is the Kruskal-Wallis test (Johnstone, Cunningham-Owens, Lawrie, *et al.*, p. 195).

36 d

(Fear, p. 343)

37 b

(Fear, p. 349)

38 b

39 d

40 e

41 a

42 b

43 d

Sensitivity = a/a + c = 228/241 = 0.95 (correct to two decimal places)

44 e

Specificity = d/b + d = 135/159 = 0.85 (correct to two decimal places)

45 a

Positive predictive value = a/a+ b = 228/252 = 0.90 (correct to two decimal places)

46 c

Negative predictive value = d/c + d = 135/148 = 0.91 (correct to two decimal places)

47 b

Likelihood ratio of a positive test = sensitivity/1 – specificity = 0.95/0.15 – 6.33

48 d

Pre-test probability = prevalence = a + c/a + b + c + d = 241/400 = 0.60

49 e

Pre-test odds = 1 – pre-test probability/pre-test probability = 0.4/0.6 = 0.67

50 d

Post-test odds = LR × pre-test odds = 6.33 × 0.67 = 4.24

51 a

Post-test probability = post-test odds/1 + post-test odds = 4.24/5.24
= 0.81

52 c

53 b

EER = c/c + d = 707/1022 = 0.69

54 e

CER = a/a + b = 684/1052 = 0.65

55 a

ABI = EER – CER = 0.69 – 0.65 = 0.04 = 4%

56 d

RR = EER/CER = 0.69/0.65 = 1.06

57 c

This question refers to the relative benefit increase (RBI).

RBI = RR – 1 = 1.06 – 1 = 0.06

58 e

NNT = 1/ABI = 1/0.04 = 25 patients

59 c

60 d

(Fear, p. 345)

61 c

62 d

63 c

64 e

65 a

(Fear, p. 345)

66 d

67 b

OR = ad/bc = 51 × 628/42 × 113 = 6.75

68 a

As the study examines events over the past week, only recall bias is somewhat minimised.

69 a

70 c

71 e

72 b

73 e

74 b

In a cohort study it is possible to calculate the relative risk.

75 c

EMIs

1 1 c

2 h

3 a

4 c

5 g

6 b

7 i

2 1 m

2 e

3 h

3 1 c

2 e

3 h

4 e

5 d

6 g

4 1 d

2 h

3 a

4 g

5 1 m

2 d

3 e

4 h

5 b

6 g

6 1 f

2 b

3 c

General adult

Questions

MCQs

1 You have started a patient with postnatal depression on an antidepressant and wish to monitor changes in her symptoms. Which of the following rating scales would you use?

   a Hospital Anxiety and Depression Scale

   b Beck Depression Inventory

   c Montgomery-Asberg Depression Rating Scale

   d Morgan-Russell Scale

   e Edinburgh Postnatal Depression Scale

2 You are referred a 62-year-old man who has an established diagnosis of Parkinson's disease, and he has developed psychotic symptoms. He has never been prescribed antipsychotics in the past. Which of the following is the best treatment for him?

   a Quetiapine

   b Aripiprazole

   c Haloperidol

   d Olanzapine

   e Risperidone

3 Which of the following is not a symptom of a temporal lobe lesion?

a Confabulation

b Impaired learning of new words

c Reduced appreciation of music

d Sensory inattention

e Perseveration

4 A 28-year-old female patient with an established diagnosis of schizophrenia has been prescribed olanzapine and quetiapine with poor effect. Which of the following options is the next step is to try?

a Clozapine

b Amisulpiride

c Haloperidol

d Lithium

e Aripiprazole

5 A man comes to your clinic nine months after the death of his mother. You find features of a moderate depressive illness. He occasionally hears her voice calling him. Which of the following is the best treatment option?

a Do nothing and reassure him it will all go away

b Start an antidepressant and follow him up

c Start an antipsychotic and follow him up

d Start an antidepressant and arrange follow-up with his GP

e Refer him for counselling

6 A patient is breastfeeding. She has bipolar affective disorder and stopped her medication before her pregnancy. She is showing early signs of relapse. Which of the following medications is safest when breastfeeding?

a Lithium

b Lamotrigine

c Sodium valproate

d Lorazepam

e Carbamazepine

7 You assess a 53-year-old woman who comes into your outpatient clinic. She is obsessed with dirt and has to wash her hands up to 20 times if she touches anything. Which of the following psychological treatments should be recommended?

a Relaxation techniques

b Cognitive-behavioural therapy (CBT)

c Cognitive-analytical therapy (CAT)

d Psychodynamic therapy

e Interpersonal therapy

8 A patient's relative comes to see you, having read about tardive dyskinesia on the internet. Which of the following is false regarding tardive dyskinesia?

a It is more common in elderly females

b It can be caused by stopping antipsychotics

c It was not described before the advent of psychotropic medication

d It is more common in patients who have affective disorder than in patients who have schizophrenia

e Clozapine is a potent cause

9 You are called to A&E to see a man withdrawing from amphetamines. Which of the following is he least likely to have?

a Insomnia

b Seizures

c Hypersomnia

d Agitation

e Decreased appetite

10 Which of the following describes a failure to recognise the whole of a complex picture but preservation of the ability to identify individual parts?

a Prosopagnosia

b Simultagnosia

c Constructional apraxia

d Visual agnosia

e Astereognosia

11 Which of the following is a recognised symptom of atypical depression?

   a Parasomnia

   b Somnambulism

   c Hypersomnia

   d Narcolepsy

   e Night terror

12 A woman comes to see you in outpatients. She has a six-month-old son, and for the last three months she has had recurring thoughts of harming him. She does not wish to harm him and these thoughts make her tearful and anxious. The birth was uneventful but she perceives it to have been traumatic. Which of the following is the most likely diagnosis?

   a PTSD

   b Postnatal depression

   c OCD

   d Baby blues

   e Puerperal psychosis

13 A 40-year-old farmer comes to see you with general malaise, poor memory, and a circumscribed 4 cm red lesion on his chest. Which of the following is the most likely diagnosis?

   a Chronic fatigue syndrome

   b Lyme disease

   c Huntington's disease

   d Hypothyroidism

   e Creutzfeldt-Jacob disease

14 Routine physical monitoring has revealed that a male inpatient who has been prescribed clozapine for the past eight months has gained 20 kg. Which of the following is the most appropriate action?

   a Switch to quetiapine

   b Switch to risperidone

   c Add sodium valproate

d Switch to aripiprazole

e Institute dietary measures and exercise programmes

15 Which of the following is a diagnostic feature of borderline personality disorder?

a Attempts to avoid real or imagined abandonment

b Depression

c Suicide

d Self-harm

e Childhood sexual abuse

16 A young man in your clinic complains of extrapyramidal side effects. Which of the following scales is best to measure the severity of his symptoms?

a Simpson-Angus Scale

b Morgan-Russell Scale

c Young's Mania Rating Scale

d Abnormal Involuntary Movement Scale (AIMS)

e Positive and Negative Syndrome Scale (PANSS)

17 A woman who gave birth to a son three weeks ago is referred to you for an urgent assessment. Which of the following is true regarding postnatal psychiatric illness?

a The severity of 'baby blues' is associated with changes in oestrogen levels postpartum

b Premenstrual syndrome is not associated with an increased risk of 'baby blues'

c Thyroid antibodies protect women against postnatal depression

d Women developing postnatal depression have double the number of life events in the preceding year

e The overall suicide rate for women in their postnatal year is markedly increased

18 You see a 63-year-old man in the A&E department who has a long history of heavy alcohol intake. Which of the following is true?

  a Total abstinence is the treatment goal of all with problem drinking
  b Those with Korsakoff's syndrome are aware of their memory deficits
  c Chlormethiazole is the drug of choice in alcohol withdrawal
  d The mamillary bodies are damaged in Korsakoff's syndrome
  e Alcohol withdrawal fits may occur up to one month after withdrawal

19 Which of the following is a feature of 'type I' schizophrenia?

  a Neurological signs
  b Thought disorder
  c Flattened affect
  d Cognitive impairment
  e Poverty of speech

20 A female patient has had several depressive episodes and one episode of hypomania in the past. Which of the following medications is best to prevent relapse?

  a Lithium
  b Carbamazepine
  c Lamotrigine
  d Fluoxetine
  e Sodium valproate

21 Which of the following is a term to describe being unable to recognise objects by palpation?

  a Finger agnosia
  b Agraphaesthesia
  c Astereognosia
  d Autotopagnosia
  e Hemiasomatognosia

22 In normal adult sleep, which of the following is true?

   a Stages 2, 3 and 4 combined give a measurement of the total slow-wave sleep

   b K complexes are seen in stage 1

   c REM sleep occupies nearly 50% of sleep

   d Theta waves on the EEG are characteristic of stage 3

   e Slow-wave sleep aids cerebral restitution

23 Which of the following are social phobias most associated with?

   a Generalising to other phobias

   b Avoidance to reduce fear

   c Obsessions

   d Compulsions to reduce anxiety

   e Depressive features

24 Which of the following has the strongest evidence base for use to augment clozapine?

   a Sulpiride

   b Haloperidol

   c Aripiprazole

   d Omega 3 triglycerides

   e Olanzapine

25 You are called to the A&E department to see an 18-year-old male who has taken cocaine. Which of the following is most likely to be true?

   a He is likely to be depressed

   b He may have bradycardia

   c He is likely to have red eyes

   d He may have respiratory depression

   e It can be detected in the urine for up to seven days

26 Which of the following is not characteristic of bulimia nervosa?
   a Self-induced vomiting
   b Severe weight loss
   c Purgative abuse
   d Feelings of self-disgust
   e Bouts of binging

27 In the outpatient clinic, you review a 27-year-old man who you
   have been treating for obsessive-compulsive disorder for the
   past three months. He has been prescribed 50 mg of sertraline
   throughout this time but has failed to improve. What is the
   preferred action at this point?
   a Increase the sertraline dose
   b Change to a different SSRI
   c Add an antipsychotic
   d Switch to venlafaxine
   e Add sodium valproate

28 Which of the following postnatal findings is the most common in
   the babies of anorexic mothers?
   a They are large for dates
   b They have lower APGAR scores
   c They are born post-term
   d They have a larger head circumference
   e They have foetal abnormalities

29 An inpatient on your ward is struggling to get to sleep at night.
   Which of the following is not a feature of sleep hygiene advice?
   a Regular bedtimes
   b A bedtime ritual
   c Avoid alcohol
   d Eat just prior to bedtime
   e Regular exercise

30 A 63-year-old male with a significant cardiac history requires treatment for a severe depressive illness. What treatment has the most evidence for depression following a myocardial infarction?

a Citalopram

b Fluoxetine

c Paroxetine

d Venlafaxine

e Sertraline

31 Which of the following is not a risk factor for neuroleptic malignant syndrome?

a Age less than 20 years

b Previous episode of neuroleptic malignant syndrome

c Female sex

d Age greater than 60 years

e High neuroleptic dose

32 Routine investigations on one of your patients reveal an elevated T3 level. Which of the following is a clinical feature of hyperthyroidism?

a Hair loss

b Weight gain

c Slowed tendon reflexes

d Loss of libido

e Bradycardia

33 Which of the following is a subtype of adjustment disorder as defined in ICD-10?

a Acute stress reaction

b Anxious type

c With disturbance of mood

d With disturbance of emotions and conduct

e With self-harm behaviour

34 Which of the following is not a recognised cause of organic hallucinosis?

   a Brain tumour

   b Caffeine withdrawal

   c Alcohol abuse

   d Poor vision

   e Hypothyroidism

35 A patient presents with a long history of alcohol over-consumption. Which of the following is not a consistent finding?

   a Raised mean corpuscular volume (MCV)

   b Enlarged liver

   c Raised albumin

   d Raised γ-glutamyl transferase (GGT)

   e Spider naevi

36 Which of the following is not one of the '12 steps' as practised by Alcoholics Anonymous?

   a Humbly asked Him to remove our shortcomings

   b Came to believe that a Power greater than ourselves could restore us to sanity

   c Made a searching and fearless moral inventory of ourselves

   d Made a commitment to accept life without the requirement of intoxification

   e Made direct amends to such people wherever possible, except when to do so would injure them or others

37 A young male patient is concerned about sexual side effects of medication. Which of the following drugs do not reduce libido?

   a Imipramine

   b Trifluoperazine

   c Diazepam

   d Risperidone

   e Carbamazepine

38 Which of the following is not associated with morbid jealousy?

   a Old age

   b Personality disorder

   c Parkinson's disease

   d Cerebral tumour

   e Hysteria

39 Which of the following is not a feature of HIV dementia?

   a Lethargy

   b Cognitive disturbance

   c Increased muscle tone

   d Increased libido

   e Incontinence

40 Which of the following is a contraindication for home detoxification from alcohol?

   a No previous history of seizures

   b Availability of an inpatient detoxification programme

   c Previous history of delirium tremens

   d Severe craving

   e No previous detoxification under medical supervision

41 You are asked to see a 27-year-old female patient in the neurological unit following a severe head injury with a post-traumatic amnesia of greater than 24 hours. Which of the following is not a common sequela?

   a Depression

   b Delirium

   c Schizophrenia-like syndrome

   d Lasting cognitive impairment

   e Personality change

42 Which of the following should not be a routine investigation for a patient who presents with symptoms suggestive of chronic fatigue syndrome?

a Full blood count

b ESR

c Thyroid function tests

d Chromosome analysis

e Liver function tests

43 Regarding the illicit drug ecstasy, which of the following is false?

a It has an effect that lasts for several hours

b It commonly causes hallucinations

c It causes neuronal serotonin depletion in animal studies

d It is a controlled drug in the UK

e It is 3,4-methylenedioxy-methamphetamine

44 Regarding solvent abuse, which of the following is true?

a It is more common among males

b Visual hallucinations are experienced by 10%

c It commonly causes physical dependency

d It usually takes place alone

e It causes death by brain damage

45 You are treating a middle-aged man who has a new diagnosis of mania. Which of the following is false?

a Antipsychotics are first-line treatments of choice for prophylaxis

b Benzodiazepines are indicated for those patients who are not adequately sedated by antipsychotics

c Double-blind trials have shown ECT to be superior to lithium for severe mania

d Approximately two-thirds of patients show a good response to lithium within a two-week period

e Sodium valproate should be considered in those who have not responded to lithium

46 A 65-year-old woman presents with depressive symptoms following a stroke. Which of the following is true?

a Depression is more common following a posterior lesion than following an anterior lesion

b A family history of depression does not contribute to the risk of depression after stroke

c Tricyclic antidepressants should not be used in depression after stroke

d Depression is thought to be more common following a left-rather than a right-hemisphere lesion

e Any depression is strongly associated with a degree of intellectual impairment

47 Which of the following has not been found to be useful in the treatment of depression?

a Pumpkin seeds

b Diazepam augmentation

c Triiodothyronine

d Lithium augmentation

e Olanzapine augmentation

48 Which of the following medications has been shown to be most effective in helping patients with borderline personality disorder?

a Olanzapine 20 mg daily

b Lithium 400 mg twice daily

c Risperidone 1 mg at night

d Moclobemide 600 mg daily

e Diazepam 5 mg twice daily

49 Regarding anxiety disorder, which of the following is true?

a Social phobia is more common among females

b Mitral valve lesions are found in over 40% of sufferers

d There is a peak age of onset in agoraphobia after the age of 50 years

d The most common change of diagnosis is to depression

e Many patients develop significant alcohol problems

50 The husband of one of your patients is keen to understand the prognosis of his wife's condition. Which of the following indicates a good outcome in affective disorder?

a Late onset

b A positive family history of depressive disorder

c Comorbid dysthymia

d Severe initial psychopathology

e Comorbid anxiety

51 Which of the following is true regarding the five-year prognosis of a patient with schizophrenia?

a 25% will remain in hospital

b 15% will have committed suicide

c Prognosis is independent of the family's response to the person

d 20% will have recovered completely

e 80% will be back at work

52 Which of the following is not a feature of LSD abuse?

a Tachycardia

b Formication

c Dilated pupils

d Synaesthesia

e Hallucinations

53 Medication contributes what percentage of total direct healthcare costs associated with schizophrenia?

a 4%

b 8%

c 16%

d 32%

e 64%

54 A pharmaceutical representative is explaining the actions of a new medication for the treatment of schizophrenia. Which of the following effects is mediated by the D_2 receptor activity of antipsychotics?

a Antiemetic effect

b Parkinsonian effect

c Weight gain

d Sedation

e Postural hypotension

55 Which of the following is not an acute symptom of benzodiazepine withdrawal?

a Convulsions

b Ataxia

c Stupor

d Hallucinations

e Rebound insomnia

56 Regarding chronic fatigue syndrome (CFS), which of the following is true?

a It develops in greater than 50% of patients with Epstein-Barr virus infection

b There are consistent abnormalities detected by functional neuroimaging

c The point prevalence for CFS is 2–3%

d Approximately 10% of patients with CFS fulfil criteria for affective disorder

e Psychiatric illnesses are a common comorbidity compared with other physical disorders

57 A patient with an established diagnosis of epilepsy presents with unusual symptoms. Which of the following features of an aura is not suggestive of a temporal lobe focus?

a Tinnitus

b Lilliputian hallucinations

c Forced thinking

d Lip smacking

e Loss of consciousness

58 Which of the following antidepressants should be avoided in pregnancy?

a Fluoxetine

b Amitriptyline

c Moclobemide

d Clomipramine

e Venlafaxine

59 You are undertaking some family work with a 23-year-old patient who has a new diagnosis of schizophrenia. What is the rate of relapse of patients with schizophrenia who discontinue medication and are exposed to a greater than 35 hours per week of high expressed emotion?

a <15%

b 25%

c 50%

d 75%

e >90%

60 Which of the following is not a recognised management strategy in treating substance misuse?

a Keeping a drug diary

b Cocaine replacement therapy

c Family intervention

d Ear acupuncture

e Amphetamine replacement therapy

61 You see a middle-aged couple who have difficulties in their sexual relationship. Which of the following is not a recognised treatment of sexual dysfunction?

a Advice

b Use of lubricants

c Use of the Masters and Johnson sensate focus techniques

d Interpersonal therapy

e Treatment of any underlying depression

62 A 29-year-old female patient with bipolar affective disorder is keen to start a family. What is the incidence of birth defects in a woman taking valproate?

a 1 in 7

b 1 in 17

c 1 in 70

d 1 in 700

e 1 in 7000

63 A patient with established depression presents with elevated mood and reduced sleep. Which of the following does not make the diagnosis of hypomania difficult?

a Recent antidepressant therapy

b Substance misuse

c Borderline personality disorder

d Symptoms of attention-deficit hyperactivity disorder

e Hypothyroidism

64 You have been asked to teach a local GP practice about the physical effects of eating disorders. Which of the following is least commonly associated with bulimia?

a Oesophageal tears

b Dental decay

c Peptic ulcer

d Parotid gland enlargement

e Seizures

65 Which of the following is the least likely psychological consequence of taking MDMA?

a Anxiety

b Disinhibition

c Increased desire to do mental tasks

d Perceptual disturbance

e Increased friendliness

66 Which of the following medications is least likely to give symptomatic relief to symptoms of social phobia?

a Fluoxetine

b Diazepam

c Buspirone

d Amitriptyline

e Propranolol

67 A GP phones you for some advice regarding a female patient who has severe symptoms of premenstrual syndrome. Which of the following is the medication of choice?

a Citalopram

b Fluoxetine

c Paroxetine

d Venlafaxine

e Sertraline

68 Which of the following personality disorders is least likely to be helped by prescription of an antipsychotic?

a Antisocial personality disorder

b Narcissistic personality disorder

c Anankastic personality disorder

d Borderline personality disorder

e Histrionic personality disorder

69 An anxious patient with an eight-month history of obsessions and compulsions is keen to learn about her prognosis. What percentage of patients with obsessive-compulsive disorder become chronic?

a 10%

b 30%

c 50%

d 70%

e 90%

70 Which of the following investigations is most likely to be seen in anorexia nervosa?

a High oestrogen

b Low cortisol

c High white cell count

d Low T3

e Hyperkalaemia

71 A 34-year-old male patient with schizophrenia refuses to take his medication in the community. Which of the following is the most common reason for non-compliance with antipsychotic medication?

a Perceived stigma

b Extrapyramidal side effects

c Lack of insight

d Complexity of the regime

e Weight gain

72 Which of the following is not a risk factor for the development of depression in multiple sclerosis?

a Female sex

b Early onset of disease

c Substance misuse

d Social isolation

e Severity of disease

73 Which of the following is true regarding the NICE guidelines for computerised CBT?

   a They were published in 2006

   b Computerised CBT should be offered to patients suffering from PTSD

   c 'Beating the Blues' was recommended for the treatment of mild to moderate depression

   d Computerised CBT should be used as a stand-alone therapy

   e There was sufficient evidence leading to the recommendation of the 'COPE' computer package

74 Which of the following is characteristic of puerperal psychosis?

   a Insidious onset

   b Significant cognitive impairment

   c Hypersomnia

   d Marked perplexity

   e Few fluctuations in mental state

75 Which of the following is not a recognised management option for somatisation disorder?

   a Supportive psychotherapy

   b Tricyclic antidepressant prescription

   c Treat secondary illnesses with appropriate psychopharmacology

   d Determine if there is an underlying medical cause

   e Limit access to multiple specialists

EMIs

1 Agnosias

   a Colour agnosia

   b Agraphagnosia

   c Finger agnosia

   d Hemiasomatagnosia

   e Prosopagnosia

   f Astereognosia

g Anosognosia

h Autotopagnosia

Which agnosias are described below?

1 Part of Gerstmann's syndrome

2 Inability to recognise objects placed in hand when eyes shut

3 Inability to recognise faces

4 Ignoring paralysis

5 Part of the body is felt to be absent

2 Treatments for opioid dependence
a Naloxone
b Urine drug screen
c Lofexidine
d Naltrexone
e Establish dependence
f Observe signs of withdrawal
g Methadone
h Buprenorphine

Which is the correct management of these situations?

1 A new patient says he takes heroin. (2 answers)

2 A patient who is well established on methadone wants a detoxification. (2 answers)

3 A patient with heroin dependence does not want to take methadone. (2 answers)

4 A patient collapses with a suspected heroin overdose.

3 Neurological signs
  a Hemianopia
  b Apraxia without alexia
  c Prosopagnosia
  d Finger agnosia
  e Ataxia
  f Pure agraphia
  g Broca's aphasia
  h Visual hallucinations
  i Perseveration
  j Wernicke's aphasia

Which of the above are associated with these?

  1 A lesion of the non-dominant hemisphere

  2 Weakness of the dominant hand

  3 A lesion of the left posterior parietal lobe

4 Adverse effects of medication
  a Neuroleptic malignant syndrome
  b Cardiomyopathy
  c Diabetes insipidus
  d Diabetes mellitus
  e Cushing's syndrome
  f Diabetic ketoacidosis
  g Delirium tremens
  h Lithium toxicity

What is the diagnosis in the situations described below?

  1 A young man on clozapine complains of breathlessness and has a persistent tachycardia.

2 A woman who has been taking steroids for her asthma is feeling low in mood. She has put on weight and has myopathy, thin skin and purple abdominal striae.

3 A young man who was started on an antipsychotic two weeks ago now exhibits stiff muscles, fever, labile blood pressure and confusion.

5 Epilepsy
   a Reflex epilepsy
   b Autonomic epilepsy
   c Gelastic epilepsy
   d Simple partial seizures
   e Complex partial seizures
   f Myoclonic seizures
   g Pseudoseizures
   h Secondary generalised epilepsy
   i Primary generalised epilepsy

Which type of seizures are described below?

1 Seizures brought on by music

2 Seizures associated with laughter

3 A patient smells flowers before losing consciousness

6 Alcohol-related conditions
   a Delirium tremens
   b Alcohol dependence
   c Korsakoff's syndrome
   d Wernicke's encephalopathy
   e Alcoholic hallucinosis
   f Alcoholic delirium
   g Alcohol withdrawal
   h Hepatic encephalopathy
   i Alcohol misuse

Which of the conditions above are described below?

1 A 44-year-old homeless man is brought into A&E. He is agitated and psychotic. The EEG shows high-voltage slow waveforms, and he is confused. There are signs of chronic liver disease.

2 A patient of yours lives in a hostel and binges heavily on alcohol on weekends. On Monday morning, staff at the hostel witness him having a seizure.

3 A woman of 55 has drunk a bottle of vodka every day for many years. She has severe problems with her memory and occasional hallucinations. She is disoriented to time.

7 EEG tracings
a Spike and wave discharge over right temporal region
b Focal delta waves
c Increased fast waves
d Triphasic sharp wave complexes
e Widespread theta activity
f Occipital alpha rhythm
g 3Hz spike and wave discharge
h General spike and wave discharge throughout the leads
i Flattened EEG
j Reduced alpha rhythm and increased beta and theta rhythm

Which is the most likely EEG tracing in these cases?

1 Huntingdon's disease

2 Creutzfeldt-Jakob disease

3 Structural brain lesion

4 Benzodiazepine use

Answers

MCQs

1 c

The Edinburgh Postnatal Depression Scale is a screening tool, but the Montgomery-Asberg Depression Rating Scale (MADRS) is sensitive to changes caused by treatment (Johnstone, Cunningham, Lawrie, *et al.*, p. 182 and p. 751).

2 a

(Taylor, Paton, Kerwin, p. 309)

3 e

Perseveration results from a frontal lobe lesion.

4 a

Patients unresponsive to two antipsychotics (one atypical) should be given clozapine (Taylor, Paton, Kerwin, p. 23).

5 b

This is the recommended treatment for moderate depression following bereavement.

6 e

National Institute for Health and Clinical Excellence. *Antenatal and postnatal mental health: clinical management and service guidance: NICE clinical guideline 45*. London: NIHCE; 2007.

7 b

CBT is recommended for OCD.

8 c

9 a

Extreme fatigue is a symptom of withdrawal from amphetamines (Taylor, Paton, Kerwin, p. 252).

10 b

11 c

(Semple, Smyth, Burns, *et al.*, p. 268)

12 c

13 b

14 e

15 a

16 a

The AIMS is used to assess tardive dyskinesia (Taylor, Paton, Kerwin, p. 71).

17 e

18 d

19 b

The other options are all features of 'type II' schizophrenia.

20 a

21 c

22 e

23 b

24 a

There is a randomised control trial supporting sulpiride augmentation (Taylor, Paton, Kerwin, p. 49).

25 d

(Taylor, Paton, Kerwin, p. 252)

26 b

A patient who is suffering from bulimia nervosa is usually in the normal weight range.

27 a

28 b

29 d

30 e

(Taylor, Paton, Kerwin, p. 167)

31 c

32 d

33 d

34 b

(Puri, Hall, p. 329)

35 c

Albumin is usually low in alcoholism.

36 d

37 e

38 a

39 d

Libido is typically decreased (Puri, Hall, p. 552).

40 c

41 c

42 d

43 b

This is not a common effect.

44 a

The most common age range is 8–19 years.

45 a

Mood stabilisers are the first-line treatment for prophylaxis.

46 d

47 b

This is specifically advised against in the *British National Formulary*. Pumpkin seeds contain natural tryptophan.

48 c

Low dose antipsychotics may be beneficial.

49 e

50 a

Early onset is a poor prognostic factor.

51 d

52 b

Formication is common in cocaine use.

53 a

(Fear, p. 279)

54 a

55 c

56 c

57 e

58 c

MAOIs are teratogenic.

59 e

As shown by Vaughn and Leff (Fear, p. 500).

60 b

(Fear, p. 489)

61 d

(Fear, p. 416)

62 a

(Taylor, Paton, Kerwin, p. 109)

63 e

64 e

65 a

66 d

(Fear, p. 245)

67 b

68 c

(Fear, p. 260)

69 b

(Fear, p. 248)

70 d

71 e

(Fear, p. 279)

72 a

Male sex is a risk factor (Fear, p. 326).

73 c

National Institute for Health and Clinical Excellence. *Depression and Anxiety – Computerised Cognitive Behavioural Therapy (CCBT): NICE technology appraisal 97.* London: NIHCE; 2006.

74 d

(Puri, Hall, p. 435)

75 b

EMIs

1 1 c

2 f

3 e

4 g

5 d

2 1 b, e

2 c, d

3 f, h

4 a

3 1 c

   2 a

   3 d

4 1 b

   2 e

   3 a

5 1 a

   2 c

   3 e

6 1 h

   2 g

   3 c

7 1 i

   2 d

   3 b

   4 j

Old age

4

Questions

MCQs

1 Which of the following is not a feature of mild Alzheimer's disease?

   a Word-finding deficits are common

   b Dyspraxia is demonstrated on drawing tasks

   c Visuospatial impairment often impairs driving

   d Focal neurological signs are common

   e There is impaired new learning

2 Which of the following differentiates late-onset from young-onset schizophrenia?

   a Persecutory delusions are less common

   b First-rank symptoms are more common

   c There are greater negative symptoms

   d Personality deteriorates quicker

   e Affective symptoms are more common

3   You are considering prescribing a tricyclic antidepressant for an
    elderly patient with depression. Which of the following is associated
    with tricyclic antidepressant prescription in the elderly?
    a   Increased postural hypotension
    b   Decreased plasma half-life
    c   Fewer anticholinergic side effects
    d   Decreased volume of distribution
    e   Increased tolerance with coexisting cardiac conditions

4   You are assessing a patient with memory problems. Which of the
    following is suggestive of vascular dementia?
    a   Gradual onset
    b   No focal neurological signs
    c   Fluctuating course
    d   Systematised delusions
    e   Early loss of insight

5   A patient asks you about the risk of problems following
    electroconvulsive therapy (ECT). Which of the following is
    associated with a poor outcome following ECT?
    a   Retardation
    b   Old age
    c   Above-average intelligence
    d   Neurotic personality traits
    e   Older age of onset of depression

6   What percentage of elderly people contact their GP in the month
    before completed suicide?
    a   5%
    b   10%
    c   30%
    d   50%
    e   70%

7 Which of the following is false regarding depression in the elderly?

a Physical illness has a significant impact on the prognosis

b 30% die within six years

c Women have a worse prognosis then men

d Having the first episode when over the age of 70 years is associated with a worse prognosis

e One in five remain chronically depressed

8 Which of the following is not suggestive of delirium?

a Abrupt onset

b Rapidly changing behaviour

c Visual hallucinations

d Variability in cognitive testing

e Preserved sleep-wake cycle

9 Which of the following is not a cause of dementia?

a Rheumatoid disease

b HIV infection

c Syphilis

d Hypothyroidism

e Systemic lupus erythematosus

10 Which of the following is consistent with Pick's disease?

a Predominantly parietal lobe damage

b Status spongiosus

c 'Balloon cells' on microscopy

d Dyscalclia

e Ventricular dilatation out of proportion to sulcal atrophy

11 You have an elderly patient with Parkinson's disease. Which of the following is true regarding the drug treatment of Parkinson's disease?

   a Early treatment with selegiline will delay the need for levodopa therapy

   b Bromocriptine acts by directly stimulating acetylcholine receptors

   c Amantadine is useful in drug-induced extrapyramidal syndromes

   d Carbidopa is a peripheral dopa decarboxylase inhibitor

   e Levodopa improves tremor more than rigidity and bradykinesia

12 Which of the following is not a risk factor for Alzheimer's disease?

   a Non-steroidal anti-inflammatory drugs

   b Down's syndrome

   c Hypertension

   d Increasing age

   e Apolipoprotein E homozygosity

13 Which of the following is true regarding normal pressure hydro-cephalus?

   a Incontinence is rare

   b It commonly presents with an affective disorder

   c It is reversible if treated early

   d CT scanning does not help the diagnosis

   e Gait is normal

14 Which of the following is not a physical complication of bereave-ment?

   a Increased serum prolactin

   b Increased adrenocortical activity

   c Increased mortality from cardiovascular disease

   d Decreased growth-hormone secretion

   e Impairment of the immune system

15 Which of the following is true of Lewy body dementia?

   a The pathology is almost identical to Alzheimer's disease

   b It affects women more commonly than it affects men

   c Visuospatial impairment is rare

   d It is a rare type of degenerative pathology in demented patients

   e It commonly coexists with Alzheimer's disease pathology

16 Which of the following drug-handling changes is increased with increasing age?

   a Total body mass

   b Gastric pH

   c Rate of gastric emptying

   d Glomerular filtration rate

   e Hepatic biotransformation

17 One of your patients is depressed and had a myocardial infarction one year ago. Which of the following antidepressants is best suited to a patient who has comorbid cardiovascular disease?

   a Amitriptyline

   b Venlafaxine

   c Trazodone

   d Citalopram

   e Sertraline

18 A carer asks you about the side effects of dementia drugs. Which of the following is not a recognised side effect of acetylcholinesterase inhibitors?

   a Nausea

   b Anorexia

   c Seizures

   d Urinary retention

   e Muscle cramps

19 Which of the following is true regarding cognitive-behavioural therapy (CBT) with older adults?

 a It is less effective in the treatment of depressive illness than it is with younger adults

 b It does not make reference to the patient's early life experiences

 c It may involve other family members

 d It is known to be equally effective with different subtypes of depression

 e It is not a suitable treatment when depression arises from actual life problems

20 You are assessing a patient who presents with memory difficulties. Which of the following is suggestive of pseudodementia rather than dementia?

 a Long history of cognitive defects

 b Confabulation

 c No insight into memory impairment

 d Dressing dyspraxia

 e 'Don't know' answers

21 A patient presents with memory problems of sudden onset six months ago with a recent abrupt deterioration. On examination there are patchy cognitive deficits. What is the diagnosis?

 a Dementia with Lewy bodies

 b Alzheimer's dementia

 c Vascular dementia

 d Pseudodementia

 e Pick's disease

22 Which of the following is not a reported benefit of acetyl-cholinesterase inhibitor prescription?

 a Improvement in neuropsychiatric symptoms

 b Reduction of time to institutionalisation

 c Lower caregiver burden

d Improvement in daily activities

e Reduction in progression of cognitive decline

23 Which of these medications has been shown to improve both retention and performance in non-demented aircraft pilots?

a Memantine

b Galantamine

c Donepezil

d Amantadine

e Rivastigmine

24 You are to arrange neuropsychological testing of a patient with dementia. Which of the following is false?

a The MMSE has a specificity of less than 60% for dementia in those aged over 65 who score less than 24

b The CAMCOG is sensitive to cognitive impairment in the early stages of dementia

c The NART can be used to estimate premorbid intelligence in those with early dementia

d The Camden Memory Test Battery tests recognition memory for words, faces and drawings

e The Wisconsin Card Sort Test should not be used in over-65s

25 A patient presents with word-finding difficulties and losing objects. There has been a gradual decline in his memory for the last eight months. He scores 20/30 on the MMSE. What is the diagnosis?

a Dementia with Lewy bodies

b Alzheimer's dementia

c Vascular dementia

d Pseudodementia

e Pick's disease

EMIs

1 Carers
   a Physical dependency in the patient
   b Living in an institution
   c Male carer
   d Male patient
   e Carer married to the patient
   f Poor relationship with the patient before the illness
   g A diagnosis of dementia in the patient
   h Living with another person

Which of the above factors are associated with:

   1 Elder abuse (2 answers)

   2 Carer stress (3 answers)

   3 A decreased risk of depression in carers (3 answers)

2 Dementia
   a Alzheimer's dementia
   b Frontotemporal dementia
   c Huntington's dementia
   d Lewy body dementia
   e Normal pressure hydrocephalus
   f Vascular dementia
   g Alcoholic dementia
   h Pseudodementia

Which of the conditions above are described below?

   1 A 73-year-old man has a pill-rolling tremor and marked sensitivity to low-dose antipsychotics prescribed for visual hallucinations.

2   A 76-year-old woman has a short history of worsening memory. She is uncooperative and inconsistent on cognitive testing.

3   A 55-year-old man has increasing disinhibition and lack of judgement. He is increasingly apathetic and inappropriate in social settings.

Answers

MCQs

1 d

There are usually no focal neurological signs (Fear, p. 448).

2 e

(Fear, p. 460)

3 a

(Puri, Hall, p. 535)

4 c

(Fear, p. 450)

5 d

Old age and late-onset depression are both associated with increased response to ECT.

6 d

(Fear, p. 459)

7 c

8 e

The sleep-wake cycle is impaired in delirium.

9 a

Rheumatoid arthritis may be protective against developing dementia, perhaps due to non-steroidal anti-inflammatory medication.

10 c

Balloon cells are not a constant feature, but are characteristic.

11 d

12 a

Non-steroidal anti-inflammatory drugs may be protective (Fear, p. 449).

13 c

A shunt can stop or even reverse the development of further dementia.

14 d

Growth-hormone secretion is increased.

15 e

16 b

(Puri, Hall, p. 534)

17 e

(Taylor, Paton, Kerwin, pp. 166–7)

18 d

Urinary incontinence is a recognised side effect.

19 c

20 e

Pseudodementia is associated with no attempt to find the answer, whereas patients with dementia often confabulate.

21 c

22 b

(Taylor, Paton, Kerwin, p. 301)

23 c

24 a

The specificity is over 80%.

25 b

EMIs

1 1   e, f

     2   d, f, g

     3   a, c, h

2 1   d

     2   h

     3   b

5

Forensic

Questions
MCQs

1 Which of these statements about arson is true?
   a All arsonists receive mandatory prison sentences or hospital orders
   b Investigation of arson usually leads to a conviction
   c Psychiatric reports should be requested in every case of arson
   d Recidivism is likely in more than half of arsonists
   e Psychosis is the most common diagnosis

2 Which of the following statements about homicide is false?
   a 9% of homicides are committed by those in recent contact with mental health services
   b Infanticide may reduce the charge from murder to manslaughter
   c 5% of homicide perpetrators have a diagnosis of schizophrenia
   d Perpetrators with mental illness are more likely to kill strangers
   e Alcohol and drug misuse contribute to 61% of homicides

3 The prevalence of psychotic disorders in male prisoners compared to the general population is approximately:

a 5 times greater

b 10 times greater

c 20 times greater

d 40 times greater

e 50 times greater

4 What percentage of sex offenders will commit a further sexual or violent offence?

a 10%

b 15%

c 25%

d 50%

e 65%

5 Which of the following is not considered when assessing fitness to plead?

a Ability to act in their own interests

b Ability to understand the charges and how they can plead

c Knowledge that they may challenge a juror

d Ability to comprehend the evidence

e Ability to instruct their solicitor

6 The association between psychosis and violence in the community is of a similar order of magnitude to the association between:

a Passive smoking and lung cancer

b Coffee and cirrhosis

c Aluminium and dementia

d The oral contraceptive pill and breast cancer

e Smoking and lung cancer

7 The mother of one of your patients is very concerned that her son will end up in prison like his father. Which of these statements about the genetics of antisocial behaviour is false?

   a Heritability of antisocial behaviour is 40%

   b Callous-unemotional traits are highly heritable

   c Low IQ is a risk factor for offending behaviour

   d There is substantial genetic overlap between adult antisocial behaviour and alcohol and drug dependence

   e Maltreated children who have a genotype conferring high MAO-A expression are more likely to develop antisocial problems than are those with low MAO-A expression

8 Which of these statements about exhibitionism is false?

   a Offenders are more likely to be married than are other sexual offenders

   b It is an indictable offence

   c Offenders are likely to display other paraphilic behaviour

   d Most convicted offenders do not re-offend

   e It is likely to occur at times of personal stress

9 Which of the following is most strongly linked to offending and violence?

   a Personality disorders

   b Schizophrenia

   c Learning disabilities

   d Alcohol and substance misuse

   e Delusional disorders

10 Which of these statements about suicides in prison is correct?

   a The rate is three times that in the general population

   b It is the most common cause of death in prisons

   c The most common method is overdose

   d Older offenders are at particular risk

   e Sentenced prisoners are at higher risk than remand prisoners

11 Which of the following is not a risk factor for a psychiatric patient causing harm to another patient?

a Persecutory delusions

b Non-compliance with medication

c Substance misuse

d Previous suicidal behaviour

e Childhood abuse

12 What is the estimated percentage of homicides that are homicide-suicide?

a 0.1%

b 0.5%

c 1%

d 2%

e 5%

13 Which of these factors is not included in the historical section of the HCR-20 risk assessment?

a Previous violence

b Response to treatment

c Relationships

d Employment

e Mental illness

14 Which of these statements about infanticide is true?

a A quarter of the mothers who commit infanticide have a mental illness

b There is a fixed sentence imposed by law

c It is a common outcome in puerperal psychosis

d The Edinburgh Postnatal Depression Scale specifically asks about thoughts of harming the baby

e It is not related to substance misuse

15 In relation to the MacArthur study of violence in the community, which of the following is true?

a The presence of substance misuse did not affect the rate of violence

b There was no relationship between mental illness and violence

c The highest rates of violence were found in those with schizophrenia

d Those with affective disorders had higher rates of violence than those with schizophrenia

e It considered only self-reported violence

16 Which of the following is true regarding shoplifting?

a It results in less than 5% of culprits being referred for psychiatric assessment

b It is a recidivist activity for the majority of females

c It is a recognised diagnosis in ICD-10

d It is a predominantly male activity

e In psychiatric disturbed patients, it is most often is due to learning disability

17 What is the age of criminal responsibility in England and Wales?

a 8 years

b 9 years

c 10 years

d 11 years

e 12 years

18 Which of the following is not classified within the ICD-10 category of disorders of sexual preference?

a Exhibitionism

b Transsexualism

c Paedophilia

d Sadomasochism

e Voyeurism

19 Regarding the interactions between schizophrenia and substance misuse, which of the following is false?

   a Substance misuse rarely manifests prior to the onset of psychotic symptoms

   b The comorbidity makes the assessment of risk of violence more complicated

   c Substance misuse is a marker for increased risk of violence

   d Treatment of substance misuse should be given a priority in reducing the risk of violence

   e Substance misuse contributes to the majority of the risk of violence

20 Regarding the treatment of sex offenders, which of the following has an established evidence base?

   a Psychodynamic psychotherapy

   b Lithium

   c Cognitive-behavioural therapy

   d Propranolol

   e Carbamazepine

EMIs

1 Risk assessment

   a Psychopathy Checklist-Revised (PCL-R)

   b Violence Risk Scale

   c Clinical judgement

   d Historical, Clinical and Risk Management Scale (HCR-20)

   e Violence Risk Appraisal Guide (VRAG)

   f ICD-10

   g Present State Examination (PSE)

   h Static-99

Which of the tools above are:

   1 Actuarial risk assessments (2 answers)

   2 Structured clinical risk assessments (2 answers)

2 Risk of offending

    a Low intelligence

    b Family criminality

    c Poor school achievement

    d Psychotic symptoms

    e Attention-deficit hyperactivity disorder

    f Poor parenting

    g Substance misuse

    h Employment

    i Asian males

Which of the factors above are:

    1 Associated with a reduced risk of offending (2 answers)

    2 Dynamic factors that increase the risk of offending (3 answers)

Answers

MCQs

1 c

It is recommended that psychiatric reports are requested as a matter of routine in arson cases (Stone, Roberts, O'Grady, *et al.*, p. 109).

2 d

Perpetrators with mental illness are less likely to kill strangers; it is more frequently a friend or family member (Swinson N, Ashim B, Windfuhr K, *et al.* National Confidential Inquiry into suicide and homicide by people with mental illness: new directions. *Psychiatr Bull.* 2007; **31**: 161–3).

3 c

The prevalence of psychosis in the influential ONS study was 7% in male sentenced and 10% in male remand prisoners, compared with 0.4% in the community (Stone, Roberts, O'Grady, *et al.*, p. 5).

4 c

Long-term follow-up of sex offenders over 22 years found that nearly a quarter committed a further sexual or violent offence (Stone, Roberts, O'Grady, *et al.*, p. 218).

5 a

To be declared not fit to plead it is not enough for the accused to be likely to act against his own interests, for example due to paranoia (Stone, Roberts, O'Grady, *et al.*, p. 56).

6 e

Maden A. *Treating Violence: a guide to risk management in mental health.* Oxford: Oxford University Press; 2007.

7 e

It is the opposite way around. Data from the Dunedin cohort suggested that maltreated children with a genotype conferring high levels of MAO-A activity were less likely to develop antisocial problems.

Caspi A, McClay J, Moffitt TE, *et al*. Role of genotype in the cycle of violence in maltreated children. *Science*. 2002; **297**: 851–4.

8 b

It is a summary offence that can be dealt with in a magistrates court.

9 d

(Semple, Smyth, Burns, *et al*., p. 645)

10 b

(Semple, Smyth, Burns, *et al*., p. 659)

11 e

12 c

13 b

Response to treatment is considered in the clinical section of the HCR-20 (Semple, Smyth, Burns, *et al*., p. 647).

14 a

(Stone, Roberts, O'Grady, *et al*., p. 245)

15 d

Monahan J, Steadman HJ, Silver E, *et al*. *Rethinking Risk Assessment: the MacArthur study of mental disorder and violence*. Oxford: Oxford University Press; 2001.

16 a

Approximately 2% are referred for a psychiatric assessment.

17 c

18 b

Transsexualism is classified within gender identity disorders.

19 a

Mullen PE. Schizophrenia and violence: from correlations to preventive strategies. *Adv Psychiatr Treat.* 2006; **12**: 239–48.

20 c

Gordon H, Grubin D. Psychiatric aspects of the assessment and treatment of sex offenders. *Adv Psychiatr Treat.* 2004: **10**: 73–80.

EMIs

1 1 e, h

   2 b, d

2 1 h, i

   2 d, e, g

6

Child and adolescent

Questions

MCQs

1   Which of the following does not correlate with an increased prevalence of mental disorders?

   a   One-parent families
   b   Families with three or more children
   c   Reconstituted families
   d   Uneducated and unemployed parents
   e   Parents who are social-sector tenants

2   Which of the following is not an ICD-10 subcategorisation of conduct disorder?

   a   Socialised conduct disorder
   b   Oppositional defiant disorder
   c   Conduct disorder confined to the family
   d   Conduct disorder, unspecified
   e   Conduct disorder confined to the school

3   Which of the following is not a recognised treatment for nocturnal enuresis?

   a   Desmopressin
   b   Reducing fluid intake before bedtime
   c   A star chart
   d   Fluoxetine
   e   An enuresis alarm

4 You are seeing an 8-year-old who has been diagnosed with hyper-kinetic disorder with no other comorbidities. What is the first-line medication that you would consider?

a Methylphenidate

b Atomoxetine

c Dexamphetamine

d Clonidine

e Imipramine

5 Which of the following is characteristic of tic disorders?

a The average age of onset is 10 years

b Phonic tics often predate motor tics

c Obsessive-compulsive disorder (OCD) symptoms occur in over 75% of cases

d Tourette's syndrome affects 1% of the population under 18

e The ratio of males to females is at least 3:1

6 Which of the following is true regarding bullying?

a Bullies are usually anxious and insecure children

b Most victims are girls

c Physical factors such as wearing glasses are by far the most common reason for being bullied

d Most victims have normal friendships

e Children with hyperkinesis are particularly likely to be bullied

7 Regarding the maltreatment of children, which of the following is true?

a Over 5% of reported cases of sexual abuse are committed by females

b Maltreatment is particularly common in the first year of life

c Having a father who drinks four units of alcohol a week is a recognised risk factor

   d Having grandparents who live in the same house is a recognised risk factor for physical abuse

   e Emotional abuse affects around 30% of children who are also being physically or sexually abused

8 Which of the following has been shown via epidemiological studies of children and adolescents?

   a Most children with psychiatric disorders are in contact with mental health services

   b 25–35% of children and adolescents have a psychiatric disorder

   c Social disadvantage is associated with a much higher rate of school refusal

   d Psychosocial disorders have become more common over recent decades

   e Delayed speech is more common in girls than in boys

9 Regarding child-onset schizophrenia, which of the following is true?

   a It is less genetic than adult-onset schizophrenia

   b Negative symptoms are often prominent

   c The onset is characteristically acute

   d Apathy and social withdrawal typically resolve faster than delusions

   e It is associated with a better prognosis than for adult-onset schizophrenia

10 Which of the following is true of Asperger's syndrome?

   a Early aloofness is more likely than in autism

   b There is marked language delay in the preschool years

   c It is also known as infantile autism

   d Marked clumsiness is more common than in autism

   e Monologues on favourite topics are common and often hard to stop

11 Which of the following is true regarding specific reading disorder?

a It is associated with small family size

b Intensive work on phonological awareness is helpful

c Audiometry should be a routine investigation

d It is present in 10–15% of children

e It is not usually associated with any arithmetical difficulties

12 Which of the following is not an indication for antipsychotic pre-scription in children and adolescents?

a The long-term treatment of Tourette's syndrome

b The acute treatment of anorexia nervosa

c The maintenance treatment of bipolar disorder

d The long-term treatment of hyperactive behaviour in learning disabilities

e The acute treatment of relapses of schizophrenia

13 Which of the following is true regarding childhood OCD?

a It was present in 70% of adults with OCD

b Psychodynamic psychotherapy is effective first-line treatment

c It affects females more than males

d Clomipramine is often beneficial

e Scan studies suggest that OCD involves temporal lobe pathology

14 Which of the following is true of solvent abuse?

a In the UK it tends to peak in late adolescence

b Two-thirds of deaths occur in children experimenting with solvents for the first time

c Deaths commonly result from status epilepticus

d Liver and kidney damage are common side effects

e 80% of associated deaths occur in males

15 Which of the following treatments reduces the frequency of enuresis?

a Atomoxetine

b Carbamazepine

c Desmopressin

d Fluoxetine

e Risperidone

16 Which of the following is true regarding anorexia nervosa in children and adolescents?

a Adequate weight gain is rarely possible without hospitalisation

b The female to male ratio is around 5:1

c Within five years 80% are fully recovered

d There is a roughly equal prevalence throughout the world

e Onset is uncommon before puberty

17 Regarding clonidine, which of the following is true?

a It is highly effective in the treatment of tics

b It is used in the treatment of depression

c It tends to make children alert and interferes with them going to sleep

d It has strong dopaminergic effects

e It may take several months for the therapeutic effects to become apparent

18 Which of the following features is not fairly common amongst autistic children?

a Hand flapping

b Hallucinations

c Echolalia

d Gaze avoidance

e Phobias

19 In family therapy, which of the following is true?

   a By definition, family rules are explicit and known to all members

   b An alliance between two family members is unhealthy

   c The focus is often on times when the problem behaviour was absent

   d Triangulation of a child with his or her parents is desirable

   e There are no randomised control trials demonstrating the efficacy of family therapy for problems in middle childhood

20 Which of the following is true regarding psychological therapies in children and adolescents?

   a 'Time out' refers to a reward for good behaviour

   b Social problem-solving skills programmes teach children to ignore their own anger in conflictual situations

   c Cognitive therapy is more effective than medication for hyperactivity

   d In behavioural therapy, rewards should be switched every few days

   e Behavioural therapy is more effective for antisocial behaviour than for hyperactivity behaviour in the long term

21 Which of the following is not a recognised cause of faecal soiling?

   a Sexual abuse

   b Fear of the toilet

   c Constipation

   d A high-fibre diet

   e Generalised learning disability

22 What treatment is not indicated for a child with hyperkinetic disorder?

   a Pemoline

   b Fluoxetine

   c Methylphenidate

d Atomoxetine

e Clonidine

23 Which of the following conditions has the strongest correlation with comorbid learning disability?

a Depression

b School refusal

c Tic disorders

d Enuresis

e Autism

24 Smoking during pregnancy is a significant aetiological factor for which condition in childhood?

a Depression

b Specific phobia

c Selective mutism

d Hyperkinetic disorder

e Schizophrenia

25 Which of the following statements about conduct disorder is false?

a Anxiety problems will substantially increase the risk of that child developing conduct disorder

b The prevalence is approximately 10%

c Having an antisocial parent predisposes children to develop it

d Peer group rejection is a common predisposing factor

e Poor prognosis is predicted by fire-setting

EMIs

1 Psychopharmacology in children and adolescents

   a Risperidone

   b Methylphenidate

   c Fluoxetine

   d Lithium

   e Clonidine

   f Clomipramine

   g Haloperidol

   h Olanzapine

   i Imipramine

   j Atomoxetine

Which medication would be the first choice in the following clinical situations?

   1. A 9-year-old boy presents with severe concentration problems, overactivity and impulsivity. His mother has noted an increasing number of simple motor tics.

   2 An overweight 17-year-old male presents with acute onset of auditory hallucinations, thought insertion and persecutory delusions. He is carrying a knife for protection and is reluctant to engage with mental health services.

   3 A 13-year-old boy presents with a three-year history of complex motor tics and vocal mannerisms, including throat-clearing. He is being bullied at school as a result of these behaviours.

   4 A 16-year-old girl has a seven-month history of low mood, anhedonia, poor sleep and weight loss, with some suicidal ideation. She has failed to respond to 18 weeks of CBT.

   5 A 14-year-old boy presents with pervasive developmental disorder with severe aggressive and violent behaviours. Behavioural therapy and environmental manipulation have not been successful in reducing his aggression.

2   Epidemiology in child and adolescent psychiatry
   a   Tic disorders
   b   Mania
   c   School refusal
   d   Specific phobias
   e   Hyperkinetic disorder
   f   Enuresis
   g   Depression
   h   Selective mutism
   i   Autism
   j   Schizophrenia

Which of the above disorders is best described below?

   1   Males have an earlier age of onset than females.

   2   The prevalence increases tenfold between the ages of 10 and
      14 years.

   3   The male to female ratio is approximately 3:1. (3 answers)

Answers

MCQs

1 b

Families with five or more children are associated with a higher prevalence.

2 e

(Fear, p. 354)

3 d

However, low-dose imipramine has been shown to be of benefit.

4 a

Formulations include Ritalin, Concerta and Equasym.

5 e

6 e

7 a

Female sexual abusers may be co-abusers with men and may be acting under duress.

8 d

9 b

Schizophrenia with onset prior to 18 years of age is typically a more severe form with higher genetic loading and pronounced negative symptoms.

10 d

11 b

12 b

13 d

SSRIs are used as first-line medication, but clomipramine is effective second-line treatment.

14 e

Males have a higher rate of death from solvent abuse, even though females are just as likely to have tried solvents.

15 c

16 e

17 e

18 b

(Semple, Smyth, Burns, *et al.*, p. 584)

19 c

20 e

21 d

22 b

(Semple, Smyth, Burns, *et al.*, p. 577)

23 e

24 d

25 a

EMIs

1   1   j

2   a

3   e

4   c

5   a

2   1   j

2   g

3   a, e, i

7

Learning disability

Questions
MCQs

1   Which of the following is associated with tall stature?
    a   Prader-Willi syndrome
    b   Williams' syndrome
    c   Klinefelter's syndrome
    d   Laurence-Moon syndrome
    e   Cornelia de Lange's syndrome

2   Which of the following statements about fragile X syndrome is true?
    a   It affects only males
    b   One of the features is micro-orchidism
    c   It is associated with a CAG repeat
    d   Adults demonstrate social anxiety and gaze avoidance
    e   It is associated with repeats on the short arm of the X chromosome

3 Which of the following is true about psychotherapies in the learning disability population?

   a Unmodified CBT can be used in the severe learning disability population

   b Guided mourning has no place in mild learning disability

   c Part of group psychodynamic therapy is progressive muscular relaxation

   d Patients with severe learning disability who have been victims of sexual abuse should be offered psychodynamic therapy

   e Cognitive techniques may be used to teach problem-solving skills

4 In Down's syndrome, which of the following is true?

   a The peak incidence occurs in children born to women aged 30–39

   b Epileptic phenomena are very rare in infancy

   c The future development of children is associated with their facial appearance

   d Receptive language function deteriorates with age

   e Children with Down's syndrome use different strategies to learn how to count from those used by 'normal' children

5 Which of the following congenital infections has not been found to be a cause of learning disability?

   a Gonorrhoea

   b Cytomegalovirus

   c Toxoplasmosis

   d HIV

   e Rubella

6 Which of the following is not a principle in the 2001 White Paper *Valuing People*?

   a Choice

   b Rights

   c Health

    d Independence

    e Inclusion

7 In Rett's syndrome, which of the following is incorrect?

    a The child develops normally until 18 months

    b The incidence is 1:30 000

    c 40–50% show self-injurious behaviour

    d It exclusively affects girls

    e It may be misdiagnosed as autism

8 Which of the following is not true of autistic disorders?

    a Core symptoms usually improve significantly with age

    b Autism is associated with fragile X syndrome

    c Onset of symptoms in childhood is required for diagnosis

    d There is a recognised association with Tourette's syndrome

    e Autism is often associated with right temporal lobe damage

9 Which of the following maternal serum markers is suggestive of a diagnosis of Down's syndrome at 16 weeks' gestation?

    a Raised α-fetoprotein

    b Lowered C-reactive protein

    c Raised chorioembryonic antigen

    d Raised human chorionic gonadotropin

    e Raised unconjugated oestriol

10 Which of the following is true following a head injury?

    a Post-traumatic epilepsy occurs in about 10% of head injuries

    b The length of post-traumatic amnesia is linked with personality change

    c Retrograde amnesia is more useful than post-traumatic amnesia in assessing prognosis

    d The onset of dementia is common when the injury is severe

    e Those with a post-traumatic amnesia of less than one hour will usually be back at work within one week of the injury

11 Which of the following is not a feature of Prader-Willi syndrome?

a Self-injury through skin picking

b Sleep abnormalities

c Frequent temper tantrums

d Hypotonia

e Insatiable appetite

12 What percentage of people with learning disabilities suffer from a concurrent psychiatric illness?

a Less than 5%

b Approximately 10%

c Approximately 30%

d Approximately 50%

e Approximately 70%

13 Which of the following is an example of tertiary prevention of disability?

a Genetic counselling

b Management of epilepsy

c Management of childhood infectious diseases

d Improved obstetric care

e Immunisations

14 Which of the following is true of offending in the learning disability population?

a Fire-setting is the most commonly committed offence

b Most offences are committed by those with borderline and mild learning disability

c Moderate learning disability is strongly associated with homicide

d Conviction for arson leads to a fixed prison sentence

e Aggression by those with severe learning disability frequently comes to the attention of the criminal justice system

15 Which of the following is commonly associated with micro-cephaly?

a Foetal alcohol syndrome

b Hydrocephalus

c Hurler's syndrome

d Down's syndrome

e Fragile X syndrome

16 Which of the following is a feature of Angelman's syndrome?

a Mild to moderate learning disability

b Smiling face

c Broad square-shaped face

d Chest-wall anomalies

e Retinopathy

17 Which of the following is incorrect regarding forensic issues in people with learning disability?

a Sexual offending is five times greater than within the general population

b In the UK there is an increased rate of people with learning disability in prison

c Arson is over-represented in people with learning disability

d People with learning disability may be less likely to conceal offending behaviour

e Opportunistic and impulsive acts are more common than within the general population

18 Which of the following is a feature of Edwards' syndrome?

a Moderate learning disability

b Alzheimer's dementia

c Broad brow

d Clenched fist

e Azoospermia

19 The prevalence of learning disabilities in the population is:

    a 0.5%

    b 1%

    c 5%

    d 10%

    e 15%

20 Which of the following statements about specific reading disorder is false?

    a It is characterised by impairment in recognising words

    b There is an increased prevalence in the other family members of an affected individual

    c The understanding of what is read is abnormal

    d It occurs in three to four times as many girls as boys

    e Omissions, additions and distortions of words occur during oral reading

EMIs

1 Developmental syndromes

    a Lesch-Nyhan

    b Prader-Willi

    c Fragile X

    d Cri du chat

    e Down's

    f Angelman's

    g Edwards'

    h Rett's

    i Williams'

    j Klinefelter's

Which of the following features are most clearly associated with the syndromes above?

1 Midline repetitive hand movements

2 Large head, large ears, hyperextensible joints, short stature and macro-orchidism

3 Somnolesence and increased appetite

4 Rocker-bottom feet and renal abnormalities

5 Hypotonic ataxia with uncontrollable bouts of laughter and epileptic seizures

6 Short stature, hypotonia, high arched palate and wide-bridged nose

Answers
MCQs

1 c

2 d

(Semple, Smyth, Burns, *et al.*, p. 709)

3 e

(Semple, Smyth, Burns, *et al.*, p. 698)

4 d

5 a

(Puri, Hall, p. 502)

6 c

(Fear, p. 380)

7 b

The incidence of Rett's syndrome is between 1:10 000 and 1:15 000 (Semple, Smyth, Burns, *et al.*, p. 711).

8 a

9 d

10 b

11 d

12 c

Overall, 20–40% suffer from a concurrent psychiatric illness, excluding behavioural problems.

13 b

(Fear, pp. 386–7)

14 b

Evidence for increased rates of sexual offending and fire-setting is based on highly selected patient samples from secure hospitals and is therefore questionable (Semple, Smyth, Burns, *et al.*, p. 645).

15 a

16 b

(Fear, p. 382)

17 b

This has been shown in the US and Australia but not the UK (Fear, p. 396).

18 d

(Fear, p. 381)

19 b

20 d

EMIs

1 1 h

   2 c

   3 b

   4 g

   5 f

   6 d

8

Psychotherapy

Questions

MCQs

1 A woman having individual psychodynamic psychotherapy with you comes in distressed, saying she has had a dream about her father sexually abusing her. Which of the following do you do?

   a Acknowledge her distress and ask her to discuss her dream with you

   b Reassure her that she has not been abused

   c Tell her you can stop her father from abusing her by contacting the authorities

   d Say nothing

   e Tell her that the dream does not mean she was sexually abused

2 A patient asks you 'What is transference?' Which of the following is the closest answer?

   a Preventing unacceptable aspects of external reality coming to conscious attention

   b Attributing one's own unacceptable ideas and impulses to the therapist

   c The reaction of the therapist towards the patient

   d The patient's feelings and reactions towards the therapist

   e Feelings of hostility towards the therapist that are expressed by harming oneself

3   Which of the following is false regarding cognitive-behavioural therapy for moderate depressive illnesses?

   a   It is most useful in those clearly showing negative automatic thoughts

   b   It has a better outcome if the patient complies with homework tasks

   c   It has been shown to be as effective as tricyclic antidepressants in several trials

   d   It is as effective as SSRI medication in socially disadvantaged groups

   e   It is not influenced by the educational level of the patient

4   Regarding group psychotherapy, which of the following is false?

   a   It is cheaper than individual forms of psychotherapy

   b   The installation of hope is a curative factor

   c   The therapist should never disclose any personal information

   d   Foulkes has been influential in its development in the UK

   e   The concept of pairing involves a new leader or idea bringing salvation to the group

5   Which of the following statements about the evidence for dialectical behavioural therapy in patients with borderline personality disorder and self-harm is correct?

   a   It is superior at one-year follow-up to CBT and treatment as usual

   b   It has no effect on incidence of self-harm

   c   It is of comparable efficacy to CBT

   d   There is no benefit compared to treatment as usual

   e   It has no effect on the number of inpatient admissions

6   Which of the following is not a feature of cognitive-analytic therapy?

   a   It was developed by Anthony Ryle in 1990

   b   The procedural sequence model is a key concept

   c   Sessions are usually for 6–12 months

d A goodbye letter is usually written

e Dilemmas, snags and traps are the three essential patterns of neurotic repetitions

7 Which of the following statements is true of Sigmund Freud?

a He was born in Salzburg

b He was related to Melanie Klein

c He wrote *Studies on Hysteria* with Wilhelm Fleiss

d He died in 1945

e He was a habitual user of cocaine

8 Which of the following concepts was originally described by Wilfred Bion?

a Projective identification

b Container-contained

c Transitional object

d Acting out

e Manic defence

9 Which of the following is not true of cognitive-behavioural therapy?

a Collaborative empiricism is used

b It is useful in pain management

c Cognitive changes generally precede behavioural changes

d Homework may be included

e Contingency planning includes consideration of internal motives

10 Which of the following is not a characteristic feature of systemic family therapy?

a Feedback loops

b Subsystem boundaries

c Circular causality

d Separation anxiety

e Homeostasis

11 Which of the following is not true of interpersonal therapy?

   a It focuses on current relationships and how these have contributed to the onset and maintenance of the presenting difficulty

   b It usually comprises approximately 16 sessions

   c It was originally developed for the treatment of depression

   d It was developed by Klerman and Weissman in the US

   e Dramatisation and games are often used

12 Which of the following is a feature of explorative psychotherapy?

   a The patient's defences are supported and reinforced

   b Medication is discouraged

   c Advice is given

   d The patient is not allowed to regress

   e The patient is discouraged from venting his or her feelings

13 During therapy, near the end of the session, a patient suddenly blurts out 'I am abusing my children' and then quickly shifts the topic to other things. Which of the following is the appropriate thing for you to do?

   a Say 'What do you mean by abusing?'

   b Keep your boundaries. End the session on time (ignoring what she has just said), and wait until the next session

   c Reassure her that everything said in therapy is confidential

   d Tell her that you have to report her to the authorities

   c Write to her GP to inform him or her

14 Your colleague asks you what has been shown to predict a good response in psychodynamic psychotherapy. With which of the following do you respond?

   a Patients without comorbidity

   b The patient's perception of the working alliance with the therapist

   c Young patients

d Intelligent patients

e The patient's perception of the illness

15 Which of the following is not a cognitive distortion as recognised in cognitive-behavioural therapy?

a Arbitrary inference

b Magnification/minimisation

c Selective abstraction

d Overgeneralisation

e Striving for superiority

EMIs

1 Group psychotherapy

a Universality

b Pairing

c Homework

d Dependence

e Fight-flight

f Cohesiveness

g Free-floating discussion

h Instillation of hope

i Interpreting transference

Which of the above factors:

1 Are curative in groups (3 answers)

2 Hinder working in groups (2 answers)

3 Are found in psychodynamic groups (2 answers)

Answers
MCQs

1 a

2 d

3 a

The presence or absence of particular cognitive errors does not seem to have any bearing on outcome.

4 c

Therapists who are open encourage the development of transference and countertransference.

5 a

Linehan demonstrated in a randomised control trial of patients with borderline personality disorder and self-harm that DBT was superior at one year follow-up compared to CBT or treatment as usual. (Linehan MM, Heard HL, Armstrong HE. Naturalistic follow-up of a behavioural treatment for chronically parasuicidal borderline patients. *Arch Gen Psychiatry*. 1993; **50**: 971–4).

6 c

CAT usually takes 10 to 12 sessions.

7 e

8 b

9 e

10 d

11 e

(Fear, p. 525)

12 b

13 a

14 b

15 e

Striving for superiority was described by Alfred Adler and refers to personality development.

EMIs

1 1 a, f, h

2 b, d

3 g, i

Index

Key: (Q) = question, (A) = answer